The ABCs *of* LUNG CANCER

The ABCs *of* LUNG CANCER

for patients and advocates

By Dusty Joy Donaldson and Kimberly D. Lester

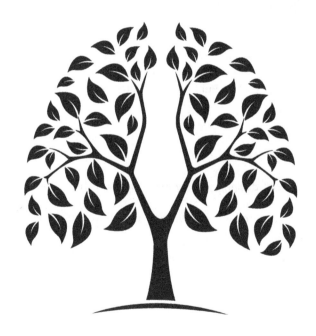

Printed by CreateSpace, an Amazon.com Company

ISBN: 1514102854
ISBN 13: 9781514102855
Library of Congress Control Number: 2016916912
CreateSpace Independent Publishing Platform, North Charleston, SC

Illustrated by Kimberly D. Lester

Cover and interior design by Dusty Joy Donaldson and Kimberly D. Lester

Tree illustration on cover from LiveLung logo created by Milan Mimmy
Kostadinovic

References and resources are listed at www.LiveLung.org/ABCs.

www.CreateSpace.com/5525870

Disclaimer

Patient advocates wrote this book. It does not include medical advice nor should it be a substitute for professional medical advice. The authors encourage patients to communicate with their doctors if they have questions about anything covered in this book.

DEDICATION

To lung cancer patients and advocates
past, present, and yet to come.

Acknowledgments

Dusty: With deep gratitude to my family, who continues to live and breathe my lung cancer journey with me.

With special recognition to my lung cancer support-group friends who helped me find my voice.

Special thanks to fellow lung cancer advocates and trailblazer friends who, by example, inspired us to believe we could actually make a difference: Bonnie J. Addario, Laurie Fenton Ambrose, Kay Bayne, Katie Brown, Chris Draft, Dr. Lynne Eldridge, Dr. Jennifer Garst, Jill Feldman, Andrea Stern Ferris, Hildy Grossman, Dr. Claudia Henschke, Cindy Langhorne, Gloria Linnertz, Karen Loss, Kimberly Ringen, Dr. Joan Schiller, and many others too numerous to list.

With heartfelt appreciation for lung cancer researchers, nurses, and doctors.

Kimberly: In addition to all of the amazing people listed above, I am so thankful to God for the gift that is my mother, that she is still with us today, and that we have been able to work on so many meaningful projects together. And I have to give a shout out to some of the rock stars of the lung cancer world: Anne Gallagher, Jessica Steinberg, Kim Wieneke, Jennifer Stauss, Linnea Olson, Lysa Buonanno, Deanna Hendrickson, Christine Dwyer, and many others. You guys inspire me. Rock on.

Contents

Dr. Eldridge, medical journalist, author, speaker, and lung cancer advocate, is the author of the National Award Winning Book, "Avoiding Cancer One Day at a Time." She is completing another book for cancer survivors titled "Keeping Cancer at Bay." In addition to speaking internationally on cancer prevention, prevention of cancer recurrence, and freelance health writing, Dr. Eldridge is a medical journalist for the New York Times Company and manages the Lung Cancer site for About.com.

FOREWORD BY LYNNE ELDRIDGE, M.D.

Whether you have been diagnosed with lung cancer yourself, have a friend or loved one with lung cancer, or just wish to educate yourself about this disease, you have come to the right place. This is not a book that will tell you which medication to use based on the specific genetic profile of your tumor. Instead, the precious nuggets contained within will help you do much more than just treat your cancer. They will help you learn how to *live* with your cancer. Dusty and Kimberly have been led to share what they've learned in over a decade as a lung cancer survivor and caregiver/advocate. A decade in which the stigma of the disease has faded, statistics have been proven wrong, and support has skyrocketed. The public is learning that, in addition to affecting men, the cancer most likely to take our mothers, sisters, and daughters is lung cancer, not breast cancer.

At this point in your journey—wherever you happen to be—you are probably all too familiar with the smoking stigma of lung cancer. I can't promise you won't hear questions about your smoking status, but reading these pages will help prepare you for the times those words are spoken. As the authors tell us, people don't ask you about smoking in order to cause you additional suffering. These comments are not usually meant to insult. In fact, these questions are often asked out of a bit of fear; people want to be reassured that they themselves are not at risk for the disease. But we know anyone with lungs can get lung cancer.

The "other" stigma about lung cancer is its survival rate. If you've missed out on the questions about smoking, you've likely been hit with one of the "other stigma" comments. For example, "My uncle had lung cancer and he only lived a few months." The face of lung cancer and the numbers describing lung cancer are changing, but it's taking time for the public to catch up. As with the smoking stigma, I can't promise you won't hear these comments, but I can promise you that the numbers that gave birth to these comments are changing. There have been a great number of advances made in both the treatments for, and survival rates from lung cancer in recent years.

Many of the numbers we use to estimate lung cancer survival are at least five years old. When I first fell in love with lung cancer survivors a decade or so ago, there was much less hope. Most conferences had only a few sessions discussing research on lung cancer. Considering that there were more new medications approved for lung cancer between 2011 and 2016 than in the 40-year period preceding 2011, those old survival numbers aren't very helpful.

Everyone with lung cancer needs support. Sometimes talking to someone who is facing the same thing is just what the doctor ordered, and the community of lung cancer survivors is alive and flourishing. (A lung cancer survivor is defined as anyone with lung cancer beginning the day they are diagnosed and for the rest of their lives.) Whether you are an introvert or an extrovert, this community of survivors is out there waiting for you. And what the lung cancer community lacks in numbers relative to other cancers, it makes up for in compassion and depth.

I can speak from experience as a breast cancer survivor who is honored to have been "adopted" by the lung cancer community. When all went well, I was surrounded by pink support. Yet when complications arose, it was my lung cancer friends who were there. These people don't flee when the going gets tough, and they hang on when the journey gets long. It's okay to be honest and raw. It doesn't matter if you've never smoked or chain smoked—those questions aren't asked. What matters is that you are a precious person deserving of compassion and care.

Dusty and Kimberly have been paving the way for those who are diagnosed with lung cancer today. The book you are holding in your hands is a treasure. It is a road map to help you navigate previously uncharted territory as a patient. These two beautiful women won't provide you with meaningless platitudes or messages of false hope. They don't mince words. Lung cancer is a challenging disease with a prognosis that is still unacceptable. By "speaking the truth in love" they share an approach which can help you move forward in an empowered way. These words can help you face challenges, prepare for the worst, but live each day to the fullest through your journey.

Aside from any words she can write, Dusty brings hope to all facing lung cancer simply by being alive. I'm often asked if I know any long-term survivors of lung cancer. Dusty and Kimberly (because they've been there) will agree that we've been in rooms with hundreds of lung cancer survivors, many who are living long term with even the most advanced stages of the disease. There is so much hope, and that hope shines beautifully through the pages of this book.

Read it. Devour it. Cherish it. Then pass it on.

Lynne Eldridge, M.D.

INTRODUCTION

For nearly a decade, we have wanted to write this book. Had we written it even five years ago, it would not have been the same book. That book would have been dark and all but void of hope. Because the world of lung cancer was dismal and hopeless.

However, the past few years have been pivotal for lung cancer. We have more reasons for hope than ever before. We look expectantly to researchers entering the field of lung cancer for new treatment breakthroughs, which are happening at an ever-increasing pace. Armies of advocates are rising to support the cause. Screening for high-risk persons is now the standard of care.

Indeed, there is a time and season for all things. Lung cancer's time has finally come. Lung cancer is still the number-one cancer killer. At least now, we have a fighting chance.

Our hope is that this book will achieve our goal of educating, encouraging, and empowering people impacted by this disease.

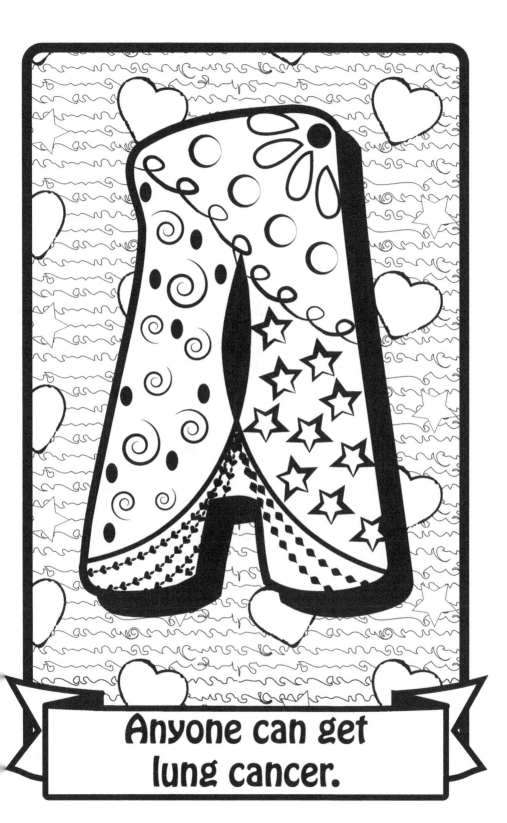

Anyone can get
lung cancer.

Jesus said,
"You're asking the wrong question.
You're looking for someone to blame.
There is no such cause-effect here."
~ John 9:3 (The Message)

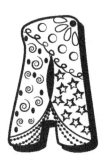

Anyone Can Get Lung Cancer

Anyone with lungs can get lung cancer. Everyone knows the number-one cause of lung cancer, but few know the number-two cause.

Many former smokers do not realize they remain at high risk for lung cancer—for life. Former smokers comprise the largest group of people diagnosed with lung cancer. This year, of the approximately 225,000 Americans diagnosed with lung cancer, half are *former* smokers. The majority of those folks quit smoking more than a decade before their diagnoses. Former long-term smokers may qualify for lung cancer screening, which significantly increases survival rates.

More importantly, whether the cause was radon exposure, smoking history, genetics, or simply a mystery, everyone is worthy of dignity and compassionate care.

Each year, more than thirty thousand Americans who never smoked will hear those four dreaded words: "You have lung cancer." In fact, more Americans who never smoked will die from lung cancer than from drunk driving, AIDS, drowning, or home fires. Although it's rare, lung cancer may even strike children.

As with other cancers, genetics can play an important role in lung cancer. Having family members diagnosed with lung cancer increases one's own risk for lung cancer.

Radon is the number-two cause of lung cancer; in people who have never smoked, it is the number-one cause of lung cancer. Radon is an odorless, invisible radioactive gas created by the naturally occurring decomposition of uranium in the soil. Radon seeps into homes. Over the course of years, it may cause lung cancer. (See "T" for information about testing your home for radon.)

People who never smoked, people who formerly smoked, and people who currently smoke can all get lung cancer. More importantly, whether the cause is radon exposure, smoking history, genetics, or simply a mystery, everyone is worthy of dignity and compassionate care. Yes, *anyone* can get lung cancer. And *everyone* diagnosed with lung cancer, regardless of the cause, deserves compassionate and equal care.

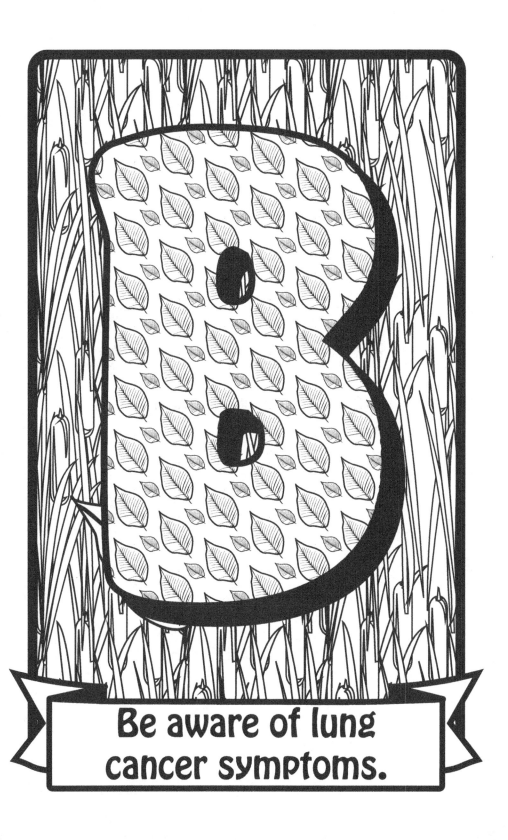

Be aware of lung cancer symptoms.

Let us not look back in anger, nor forward in fear, but around in awareness.
~ James Thurber

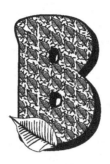

Be Aware of Lung Cancer Symptoms

Being aware of lung cancer symptoms can contribute to early diagnosis and lead to a better outcome. It is especially important for those with a history of smoking to know lung cancer warning signs. It is also wise for people who have never smoked to be knowledgeable. Knowing the symptoms may not only help you; it may also help your loved ones. When people do not fit the stereotype for someone at high risk for lung cancer, they may mistakenly dismiss classic lung cancer symptoms. Patients may go through round after round of antibiotics, only to learn they wasted precious time. Keep in mind that each year, tens of thousands of Americans who have never smoked are diagnosed with lung cancer. Former smokers may also mistakenly believe they are immune to lung cancer. As we mentioned previously, half of new diagnoses are in former smokers.

Knowing the symptoms may not only help you; it may also help your loved ones.

Every person is different. Rarely will someone experience all the symptoms. Many experience no symptoms. The following are the most common symptoms of lung cancer:

- Persistent coughing
- Persistent tickle in throat
- Persistent and extreme tiredness

- Shortness of breath
- Coughing up blood
- Changes in voice (loss of voice, raspy voice, hoarseness)
- Wheezing
- Repeated lung infections, such as pneumonia or bronchitis
- Pain in the chest, shoulder, or back (unrelated to an injury)
- Unexplained weight loss
- Swollen or enlarged lymph nodes
- Headaches, bone pain, or other unexplained pain (if the cancer has spread to other body parts)

Early detection is key to increasing survival chances. Often, early-stage lung cancer has no symptoms until the disease has spread. Knowing the symptoms of lung cancer is good. Nevertheless, screening is better. (See "E" for more information about screening.) Do not ignore lung cancer symptoms. Be smart. Be aware.

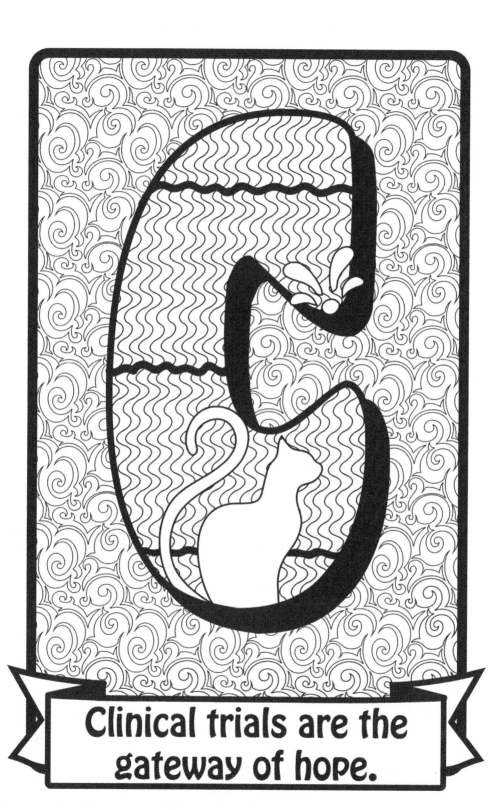

Clinical trials are the gateway of hope.

People are not for clinical trials.
Clinical trials are for people.
~ Richard Pazdur

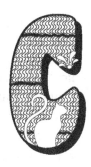

Clinical Trials Are the Gateway of Hope

Lung cancer patients are entering promising clinical trials in ever-increasing numbers. Yet the need for more lung cancer patients to enter trials is greater than ever. As additional lung cancer patients enter clinical trials, treatment options—along with survival rates—improve.

Smart lung cancer patients understand that clinical trials are at the very heart of cutting-edge scientific breakthroughs. Some lung cancer patients are thoroughly knowledgeable in how clinical trials function. These patients follow treatment plan A; if that fails, they move on to plan B, and so on, based on the latest trials underway. They enter one clinical trial after another, searching for the latest scientific advancement to help them live longer, better lives.

As more lung cancer patients enter clinical trials, treatment options— along with survival rates—improve.

Other patients may enter a clinical trial only after they have exhausted all other treatment options. There are also some reluctant patients who mistakenly equate entering a clinical trial with being a guinea pig or lab rat.

According to the National Institutes of Health, clinical trials are research studies that explore whether a medical strategy, treatment, or device is safe and effective for humans. A clinical trial is one of the final stages of a long and careful research process.

Ultimately, the goals of clinical trials are to determine if a new treatment (A) improves patient outcomes, (B) offers no benefit, or (C) causes unexpected harm. Even if the trial offers no benefit or causes unexpected harm, scientists learn and build on that knowledge. Only after courageous lung cancer patients entered clinical trials were the standard treatment options we have today approved for our use.

Whether you are depending on clinical trials for your plans A–Z or a clinical trial is your last hope, be encouraged knowing that not only are you helping yourself, you are also helping others by ultimately advancing medical knowledge to improve patient care.

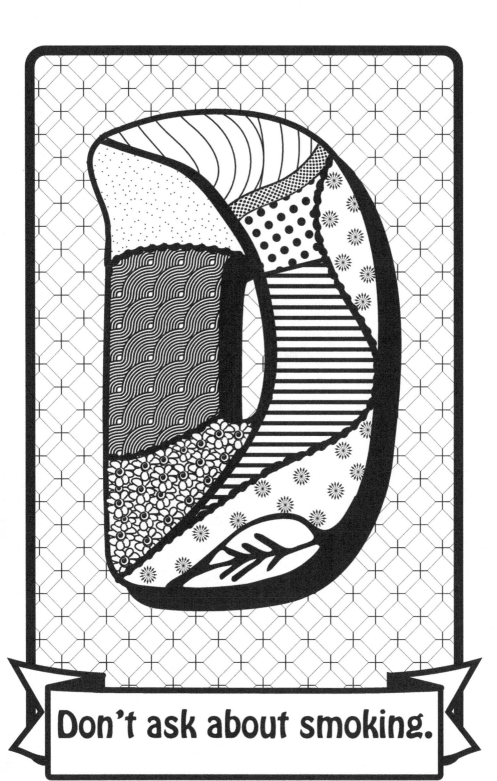

Don't ask about smoking.

If you judge people,
you have no time to love them.
~ Mother Teresa

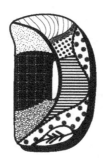

Do Not Ask, "Did You Smoke?"

"Did you smoke?" is perhaps the most common response people diagnosed with lung cancer receive. Anyone diagnosed with lung cancer knows there is a stigma with this disease that most other cancers or diseases do not have. If someone says he or she has breast cancer, the most natural response is a compassionate embrace or kind words. With lung cancer, though, the most common response is that question: "Did you smoke?" The question implies the patient brought the disease upon him- or herself. This is similar to the stigma that accompanies AIDS. In addition to inflicting unnecessary angst and emotional injury, the stigma of lung cancer has created an apathetic culture that has resulted in lung cancer research being shamefully underfunded.

This is not the time to judge, criticize, or condemn a person with lung cancer, nor is it the time for bitterness, resentment, or punishment toward someone who smoked.

This is not the time to judge, criticize, or condemn a person with lung cancer, nor is it the time for bitterness, resentment, or punishment toward someone who smoked. Considering lung cancer's dismal mortality rate, the last thing that person needs is an accusation or judgmental response to their diagnosis.

It's simple: be kind. If you don't know what to say, try

something like this: "I am so sorry to hear this. You will be in my thoughts and prayers. I am here for you if there is anything I can do."

Everyone deserves compassionate and quality care, regardless of his or her smoking history. You now are enlightened. Enlighten others.

For those diagnosed with lung cancer, try to understand that people who ask you this question do not intentionally mean to cause you additional suffering. Be patient. Try not to take it personally. One lung cancer advocate came up with a thoughtful response: "Why do you ask?" Or you can use your response as an opportunity to educate the person. "Yes, I was a smoker. I quit twenty-five years ago. After my diagnosis, I was surprised to learn that nearly two-thirds of new lung cancer diagnoses are in former smokers or people who never smoked."

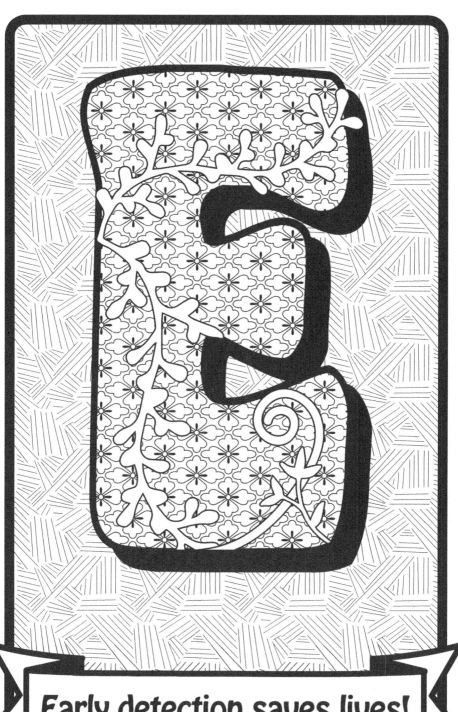

Early detection saves lives!

Early detection saves lives.
~ Science

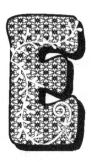

EARLY DETECTION SAVES LIVES

We have known this about other cancers. Finally, science proved what common sense has told us about lung cancer all along: lung cancer screening saves lives. In fact, lung cancer screening promises to save more lives than any other type of cancer screening. The earlier lung cancer is caught, the better a patient's chances for survival—and the better the chances for a cure. The National Lung Screening Trial showed that with annual low-dose CT scans, those at high risk for lung cancer had 20 percent fewer deaths than those screened by chest x-ray. Based on that study, the US Preventive Services Task Force now recommends annual low-dose CT scans for those at high risk. In general, the minimum age for screening is fifty-five, and the minimum smoking history is thirty pack years. Calculate pack years by multiplying the average packs of cigarettes a patient smoked each day by the number of years the patient smoked. For example, a person who smoked two packs a day for fifteen years has a thirty pack-year smoking history. (In some instances, if there is an additional risk factor, such as a family history of lung cancer or radon exposure, a different set of guidelines set by the National Comprehensive Cancer Network

Finally, science proved what common sense told us all along: lung cancer screening saves lives.

lowers the minimum age to fifty and the minimum pack years to twenty.) Former smokers who meet these guidelines may also qualify if they quit within the past fifteen years.

People often ask why not everyone can be screened for lung cancer. That is a fair question. For high-risk people, screening benefits outweigh screening risks. It is important to understand, however, that there are risks, even with low-dose CT scans. Radiation exposure is relatively low, compared with other CT scans, but exposing healthy people who are at low risk for lung cancer to radiation year after year could actually *cause* lung cancer.

While screening significantly increases survival rates for people at high risk, it's simply not for everyone. Screening does not help people who do not meet age and smoking history guidelines. However, researchers are diligently trying to find another safe method of detecting lung cancer early—for everyone. For, as we know, anyone can get lung cancer.

In the meantime, help get the word out about screening for those who do meet the guidelines. When detected early, lung cancer can be cured. If someone you care about meets the criteria for lung cancer screening, encourage him or her to be screened. (See "X" for more information.)

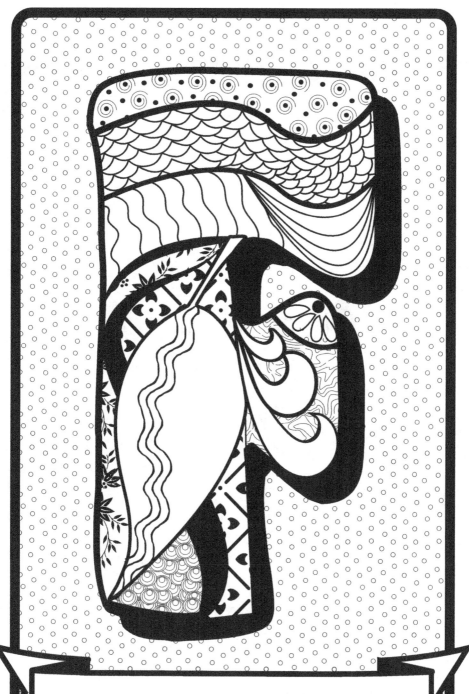

Forget the statistics!

facts are stubborn things,
but statistics are pliable.

~ Mark Twain

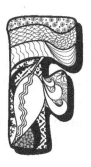

FORGET THE STATISTICS

We have a conundrum. We want to shock the world with uncommon lung cancer facts without instilling fear or discouragement in our friends fighting this disease. We also do not want to be dismissive of the seriousness of this life-threatening disease. Make no mistake: lung cancer is the number-one cancer killer.

There is a time to know lung cancer facts and understand the statistics. There is also a time to forget those facts.

The sad truth is that lung cancer statistics are dismal. However, understanding the seriousness of this disease does not mean losing hope.

Frankly, there has not been a better time to be diagnosed with lung cancer. Do not allow the disheartening numbers to overshadow breakthroughs in diagnosis and treatment. Targeted therapy, screening, robotic surgery, and precision radiation are just a few medical advances that offer the promise of dramatically changing outcomes for those with a lung cancer diagnosis. At this very moment, researchers are diligently searching for more lifesaving breakthroughs. (See "H" for more about hope.)

The lyrics of a song made popular by the band the Byrds in the

1960s actually originated from Solomon in the book of Ecclesiastes. They capture the heart of our message here: "There is a time for everything and a season for every activity under the heavens" (Ecclesiastes 3:1). In that spirit, there is a time to know lung cancer facts and understand the statistics. There is also a time to forget those facts. If you are fighting against the odds, forget the statistics.

If you are the kind of person who struggles to forget the statistics, try focusing on the fact that out of every one hundred people diagnosed with lung cancer, nearly eighteen people will survive. You could be one of those survivors. Surviving a lung cancer diagnosis is challenging—not impossible. After all, every year, more than thirty-six thousand lung cancer patients celebrate reaching their five-year survival mark. Why not you?

While lung cancer survivors are more precious than silver and gold, there is an ever-increasing number of long-term survivors. Many share their stories online. Let them inspire you to be numbered among other longtime lung cancer survivors.

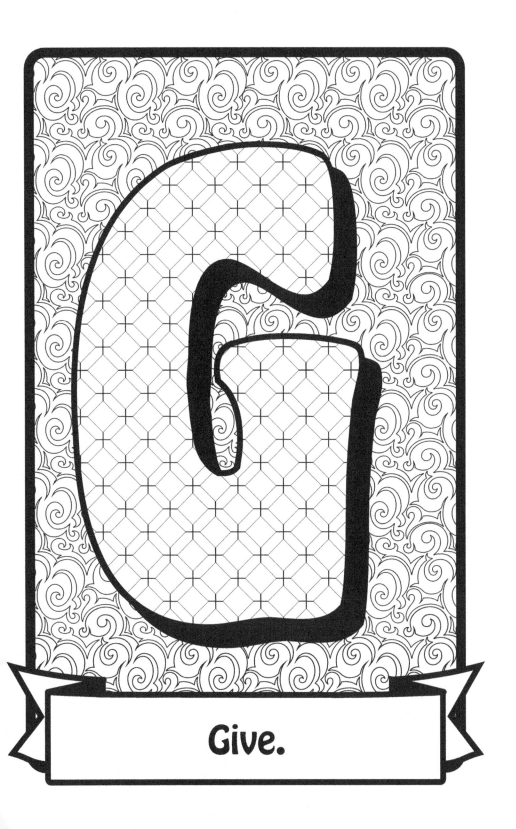

Give.

We make a living by what we get,
but we make a life by what we give.
~ Winston Churchill

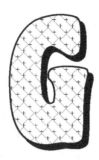

Give Something—Anything—to Support the Cause

Everyone has something to give, and this cause needs *everyone's* support. Here's why.

Frankly, because lung cancer is the number-one cancer killer, the lung cancer community does not yet have the army of survivors that other cancers have. Add the stigma of this disease to that fact, and you can appreciate how much we need advocates with the strength, courage, and resources to advance this cause.

Allow others the pleasure of demonstrating their support. It will give them true purpose and deep gratification.

Let me be clear about this: lung cancer patients—especially those undergoing treatment—please do not feel obligated to do anything. You are in the trenches, fighting this disease. However, you can delegate responsibility to the folks surrounding you. Chances are they are offering to do something—anything—to help. Allow others the pleasure of demonstrating their support. It will give them true purpose and deep gratification.

Survivors out of treatment who are otherwise healthy should give serious thought to how they can help others less fortunate than themselves. The simple fact that you survived offers hope and encouragement to others who desperately need it. Share your story freely.

There are countless ways to support the cause of lung cancer advocacy. Often the most talented people are also the busiest. The most practical way for them to give may be financially. Instead of money, people experiencing financial hardship after a lung cancer diagnosis may be able to give more of themselves, such as by sharing their story. Some people are gifted organizers. Some people have a gift of time to give. Here are a few suggestions to consider how you may best help:

- Speak to your neighbors, friends, and relatives about the need for compassion.
- Speak to your senator or congressperson about the need for increased lung cancer research funding.
- Volunteer for a lung cancer awareness/fund-raising event in your community.
- Better yet, organize a lung cancer awareness/fund-raising event in your community.
- Make a donation or fund-raise for a nonprofit organization focused exclusively on lung cancer.
- If a loved one dies from lung cancer, consider that you may make a charitable donation to a lung cancer advocacy organization "in lieu of flowers."

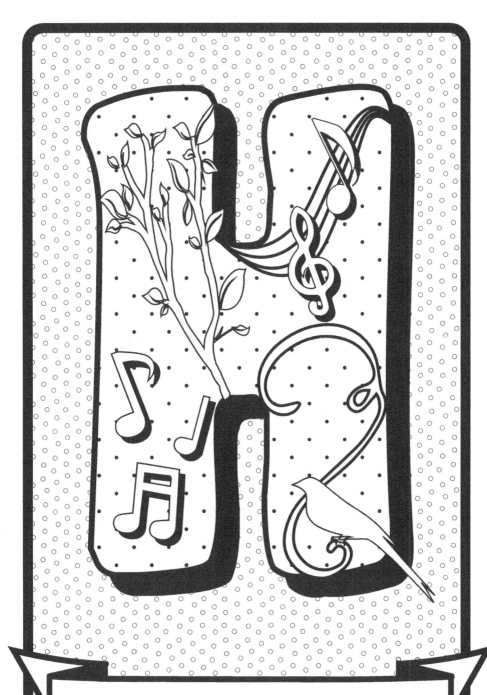

Hope

Hope is a thing with feathers
that perches in the soul and
sings the tune without the words
and never stops...at all.
~ Emily Dickinson

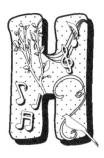

HOLD FAST TO HOPE

Hope takes many shapes and is as unique as people are. We may hope for a cure, another treatment option, or just another day. We have known lung cancer patients who had very grim prognoses hold fast to certain hopes or expectations. To everyone's amazement, they live to celebrate that special wedding anniversary, attend their son's graduation, or walk their daughter down the aisle.

Our hopes and aspirations change, depending on where we are in life and in our lung cancer journey.

Over time, our hopes change. The hopes and dreams of a newly married couple may be to one day have children. Later in their life, their hopes may be for their children to go to college and succeed. In their retirement years, their hopes may be to maintain their independence and remain in their home.

Likewise, as lung cancer patients, our hopes and aspirations change, depending on where we are in life and in our lung cancer journey. Some hope and believe for nothing short of a miracle—because it would take nothing less than a miracle to survive. Others hope that their treatment continues to keep cancer at bay. Still others hope they will make peace with loved ones before their final time comes.

Lung cancer patients and advocates have more reason to hope than ever before. Several scientific developments point to a very promising future for people with lung cancer. In fact, many patients are reaping the benefits of recent improvements in lung cancer treatments.

Much of our hope lies in medical research. Historically, lung cancer research has been shamefully underfunded. We are entering a new era for lung cancer research funding. Evidence of this is the 2013 Recalcitrant Cancer Research Act, which requires the National Cancer Institute to develop a scientific research model to address lung cancer. In addition, many nonprofit lung cancer organizations and pharmaceutical leaders are funding lung cancer research.

Lung cancer screening also offers great hope for early detection, which leads to significantly improved survival rates. Clinical trials are another cause for hope. Many long-term lung cancer survivors credit clinical trials with their survival. We could fill books with more about targeted therapy and other promising breakthroughs that scientists are pursuing. Finally, we are making incremental progress in dispelling the stigma of this disease. While there is much more to be done, every day brings a new reason for hope.

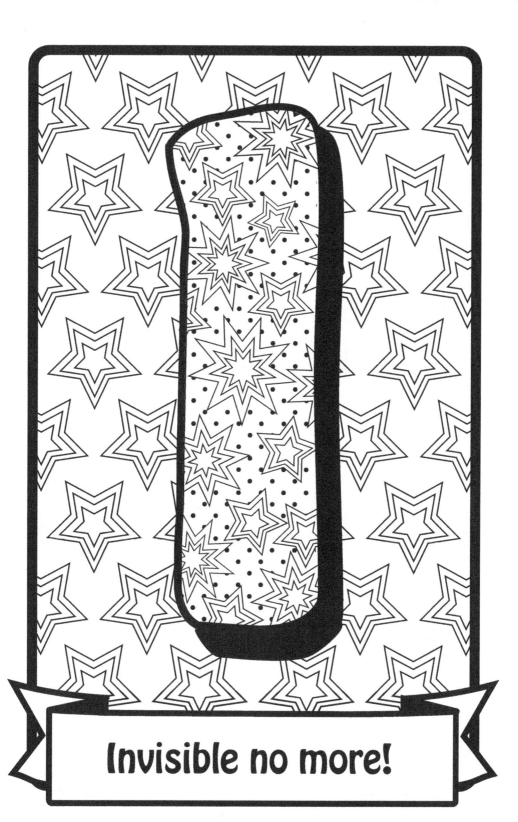

Invisible no more!

faith has to do with things
that are not seen and
hope with things
that are not at hand.
~ Thomas Aquinas

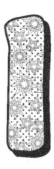

INVISIBLE NO MORE

Most cancers have an awareness month and a color. For example, the most recognized color is the pink ribbon, representing breast cancer. In October, Breast Cancer Awareness Month, the world is awash in pink! November is Lung Cancer Awareness Month. However, what color represents lung cancer? The answer to that question is not as straightforward as with other cancers because lung cancer's "color" is actually clear. How does one color something clear?

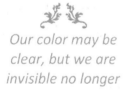

Our color may be clear, but we are invisible no longer

This issue has frustrated lung cancer advocates for years. Some use white instead. Some use pearls to represent lung cancer. Some lung cancer organizations adopted teal as their color, even though that color represents ovarian cancer.

For decades, lung cancer has been the number-one cancer killer. Lung cancer also has been the least funded major cancer in terms of federal research dollars. Couple those facts with the clear color for lung cancer, and it is easy to understand why the lung cancer community felt as if their cause was as invisible as their color.

An old proverb says that you cannot know where you are going unless you know where you have been. For people new to lung cancer or the lung cancer advocacy movement, it is important to understand the dramatic changes in the world of lung cancer in recent years.

Until December 2013, there was no early detection protocol for lung cancer. Not until a patient's symptoms developed did diagnostic tests start. Unfortunately, more often than not, by the time symptoms appear, the cancer has already spread. Thankfully, now we can catch lung cancer early through screening for those at high risk.

Another measure of success in the world of lung cancer is treatment. Until recent years, the treatment for lung cancer comprised the same chemotherapy agents used for decades. There had been few to no advances to improve treatment. Now we have several targeted agents that may significantly extend life as well as improve the quality of patients' lives.

In 1995, there was only one advocacy organization dedicated exclusively to lung cancer, Lung Cancer Alliance. In 2005, there were still precious few advocacy organizations serving the lung cancer community. There are dozens now, giving the lung cancer community a strong voice.

Yes, lung cancer is still the number-one cancer killer. And it remains severely underfunded. However, lung cancer is now on a trajectory that promises positive change. Our color may be clear, but we are invisible no longer. Lung cancer's time has finally arrived!

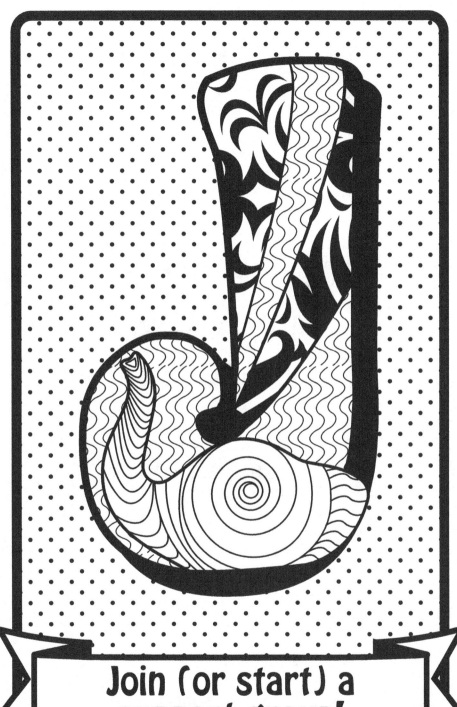

Join (or start) a
support group!

When we tell our stories
in a safe community,
all those things that separate us
go away.
~ Sarah Markley

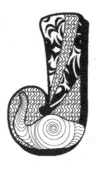

Join (or Start) a Support Group

People diagnosed with lung cancer face all the challenges as people with other types of cancer, but they often also face judgment, stigma, and isolation. After my own diagnosis, I felt that isolation, even though friends and family surrounded me. I really wanted to meet other lung cancer patients and learn from their experiences.

We all have something very important in common: lung cancer.

Some people think that a support group is where people get together to cry and feel sorry for each other. Sure, there may be tears, especially when a group loses one of its members, but the support groups I have been part of are full of life and laugher. We share stories and learn from each other's experiences. We also have speakers, such as pulmonologists, oncologists, nurse navigators, and oncology fitness and nutrition experts, as well as inspirational messages from survivors. During each meeting, everyone shares updates about his or her journey. Sometimes we simply get together for a cookout or a holiday celebration. We develop lifelong friendships. We have men and women of various faiths, political persuasions, and cultures. We all have something very important in common: lung cancer.

As important as lung cancer support groups are, there are only about one hundred in the United States. Historically, social workers and nurses facilitated support groups. Because it is unlikely they have time to take on this additional responsibility, it is unrealistic to expect significant increases in the number of professionally led lung cancer support groups. However, another way to meet the need is by engaging lung cancer survivors and advocates to facilitate meetings in their communities. Nurse navigators regularly attend our meetings and help with patients' medical questions and concerns that may arise. While they may not have the time to organize regular meetings, they are much more likely to participate in a meeting planned by others and offer their support to the support group. This model of peer-led lung cancer support groups will help reach those who may have no other support system. I regularly attended monthly lung cancer survivor meetings for eight years in a nearby town before starting one in my town. Now, part of the mission of our nonprofit is helping others start lung cancer survivor or support groups in their own towns.

If there are no support groups in your community, and you are not able to start one, get connected with others online (visit LiveLung.org for more information).

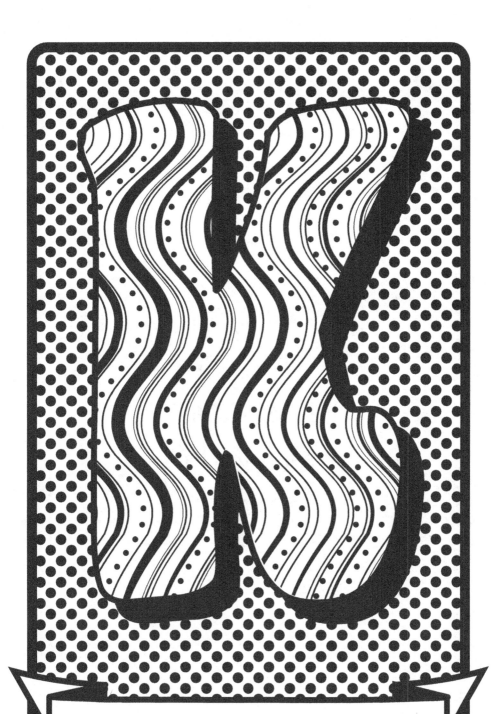

Know lung cancer facts.

Know thy self,
know thy enemy.
A thousand battles,
a thousand victories.

~ Sun Tzu

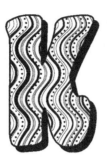

KNOW THE FACTS ABOUT LUNG CANCER

Knowledge is power. To be an effective advocate—even for yourself—you need to know basic lung cancer facts. As we discussed previously, be forewarned, not discouraged. As a patient, take heart knowing that armies of advocates are fighting on your behalf. Understanding the seriousness of this disease is important for patients, loved ones, and advocates. Brace yourself. Here are the cold, hard facts:

Understanding the seriousness of this disease is important.

- Lung cancer is the number-one cancer killer of both men and women in the United States and worldwide. Lung cancer kills nearly twice as many women as breast cancer and three times as many men as prostate cancer. In fact, lung cancer kills more people than breast, colon, prostate, and pancreatic cancers combined.
- In spite of lung cancer being the deadliest cancer, it is the least funded of all major cancers in terms of federal research funding. One reason for the lack of lung cancer research funding is the stigma associated with this disease.
- Radon, an odorless, invisible radioactive gas, is the number-two cause of lung cancer. In people who never smoked, radon is the number-one cause of lung cancer.

- Lung cancer screening for those considered at high risk can reduce the mortality rate by 20 percent or more.
- Approximately 17 percent of lung cancer patients survive five years. To put that in context, consider survival rates for other major cancers: the survival rate for breast cancer is 90 percent; for colon cancer, 65 percent; and for prostate cancer, 99 percent.

These facts speak for themselves. No one should take a lung cancer diagnosis lightly. Rather than parroting empty platitudes about beating cancer with a positive attitude, we believe in speaking truth in love. A positive attitude is wonderful—whether or not you are fighting cancer. Putting unrealistic expectations on patients is simply not fair. It is likely to do no more than add to their stress and anxiety. Cancer patients—and especially lung cancer patients—should not feel guilty for having normal feelings of highs and lows. Now, go back and read the message under the letter "F."

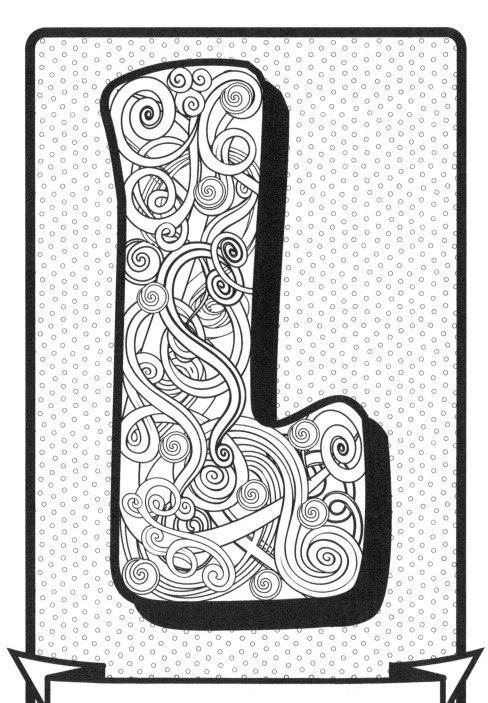

Live. Laugh. Love.

Go confidently in the
direction of your dreams!
Live the life you've imagined.
~ Henry David Thoreau

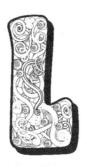

LIVE! LAUGH! LOVE!

This is good advice for everyone. How much more should lung cancer patients embrace these three simple words? Live your life as if it is the only one you have. Because, guess what? It is. We have seen very ill lung cancer patients work full time until the day they died—literally. If your job brings you joy and fulfillment, then work. If your job brings you stress and saps all your energy, leave it—if at all possible. Maybe your employer

Everyone's days are numbered. Learn to live, laugh, and love every day.

offers short-term or long-term disability leave. Doctors understand the seriousness of a lung cancer diagnosis and treatment and are usually happy to authorize your disability documents. Patients with advanced lung cancer can usually be fast-tracked for approval of Social Security disability benefits.

No one knows when one's time will come. A lung cancer friend once asked her oncologist how much time he thought she had. She was diagnosed in the spring. He told her she most likely would not live to see Christmas. Ironically, the oncologist unexpectedly died in a car accident. However, my friend lived to see nine Christmases.

Everyone's days are numbered. Learn to live, laugh, and love every day. Here are a few suggestions to live your life with abandon:

- Take a cruise. Go on a victory cruise when you complete treatment or reach a treatment landmark.
- Get a massage. It may last only an hour, but it will be one of the most relaxing hours you have ever experienced.
- Order dessert. If you're too full to eat it, take it home and enjoy it later.
- Enjoy a girls' weekend or a weekend with the boys.
- Get away for a few days—alone.
- Allow loved ones to get closer to you.
- See a Broadway show.
- Buy a new outfit.
- Forgive.
- Eat well.
- Volunteer.
- Make a bucket list. Do something on it today!

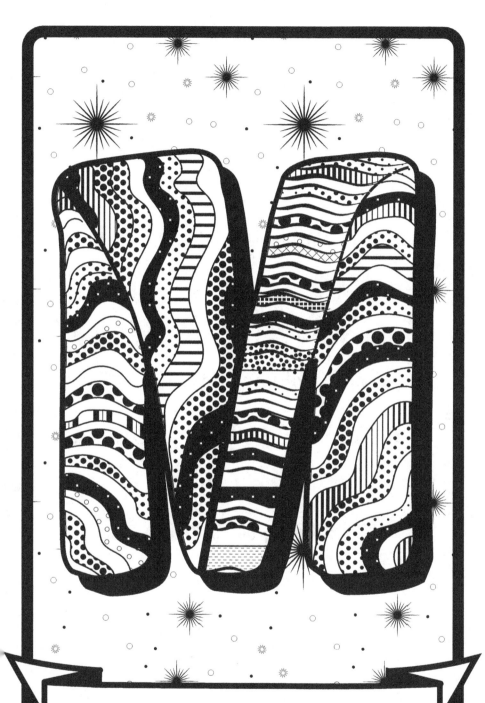

Make your wishes known.

A man may have a hundred children and live many years; yet no matter how long he lives, if he cannot enjoy his prosperity and does not receive proper burial, I say that a stillborn child is better off than he.

~ Solomon, Ecclesiastes 6:3

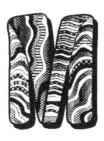

MAKE YOUR WISHES KNOWN

This may be difficult for some to hear. Nevertheless, it must be said. There comes a day for every person, whatever his or her faith (or lack thereof), to depart this life. Consider how you will leave. Will your children or spouse have to make excruciatingly difficult decisions on your behalf during raw, emotional grief? Will your arrangements cause division among loved ones who are second-guessing your wishes?

Every responsible adult has a duty to make decisions about his or her final arrangements and let others know. How much more important is this for someone with lung cancer?

Every responsible adult has a duty to make decisions about his or her final arrangements and let others know. How much more important is this for someone with lung cancer?

On a personal note, after my diagnosis, I refused to go into surgery until I had made all my arrangements. I had documents prepared for a health-care power of attorney and clear instructions on whether to resuscitate. I updated my last will and testament. Later, I also purchased a burial plot and selected some music for my funeral.

Recently, my eighty-three-year-old mother handed me her handwritten obituary. She worded it beautifully. When her time comes, my mother's obituary will say exactly what she wanted. For those of us who love her, that is a precious gift.

Making arrangements does not mean you are giving up. It is actually a way to demonstrate command over your life. Write your wishes down. Tell your loved ones. If you are in a position to do so, pay for your burial or cremation in advance.

Preparing in advance is an act of love that will spare your loved ones undue stress at the most difficult of times.

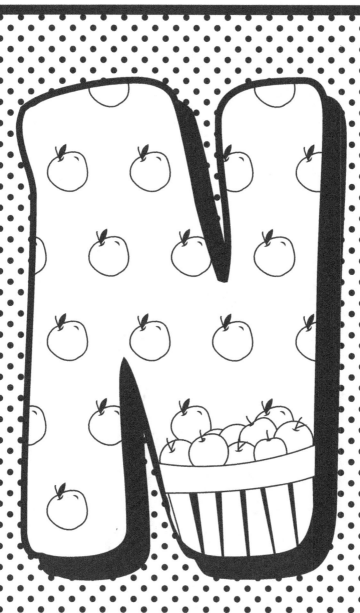

Nutrition matters!

All you need is love.
But a little chocolate now and then
doesn't hurt.
~ Charles Schulz

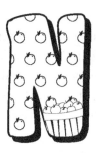

Nutrition Matters

Anyone who has been diagnosed with lung cancer can tell you, if there is one area in which you can expect to be ambushed with well-meaning advice, it's nutrition. Intelligent, level-headed friends will thrust books on questionable herbal juice cures into your hands. Everyone with your e-mail address will forward information on the latest cause or cure for cancer.

At a time when so many things feel out of control, your diet might be one thing you can control.

What you choose to eat is one of the most personal choices you can make. At a time when so many things feel out of control, your diet might be one thing within your control. You may welcome some of this advice, or you may be skeptical. You may choose to go meat-free and juice fresh veggies every morning. On the other hand, you may choose to let go of any previous restrictions you had on your diet and embrace eating the foods you enjoy.

Alternatively, you may find that whichever path you choose, your tastes, cravings, and appetite have changed because of the cancer or treatment. Cancer can change the way your body absorbs nutrition from your food as well. It is important to make sure your body is getting what it needs. Restricting calories is often not the healthiest choice for those fighting cancer.

Whatever your personal food choices may be, be gentle with yourself. It's true that some foods have cancer-fighting properties, but it's also true that a diet of brussels sprouts and garlic may not be worth living for. Eating familiar, comforting foods may help nourish you in ways that so-called healthy foods may not. Remember that what you eat can greatly affect how you feel as well as your energy levels. Try to find the balance that works well for you. Whether you choose to indulge or not, try to give your body—and your soul—the nourishment it needs to be the best it can be.

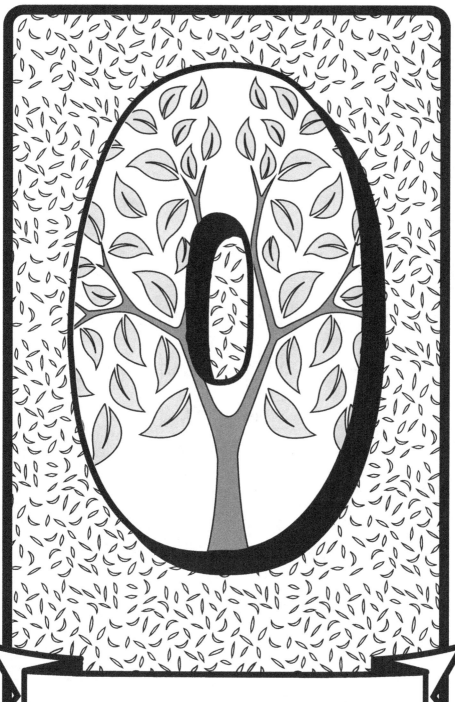

Opinions: 2 are better than 1!

He cannot be a useful counselor who
will hear no opinion but his own.
~ Samuel Johnson

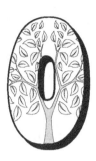

OPINIONS: TWO ARE BETTER THAN ONE

As we discuss elsewhere, dynamic scientific advancements are transforming lung cancer treatment at a faster rate than ever before, challenging even the brightest and most caring doctors to keep current.

Even if you have full confidence in your doctor, consider obtaining a second opinion. A patient's request for a second opinion will not threaten a competent and confident doctor. If it does, you may not only need a second opinion—but a different doctor.

A patient's request for a second opinion will not threaten a competent and confident doctor.

When deciding where to go for a second opinion, be sure to go outside your current doctor's facility or network. You may need to travel to get an opinion from a highly ranked facility, such as a National Comprehensive Cancer Center. Ask others on their own lung cancer journeys or ask friends if they know people willing to share their experiences with different oncologists and facilities.

Some people are so eager to start treatment that they are reluctant to seek a second opinion because of the added stress of delaying treatment while scheduling yet another doctor visit and obtaining medical records. If obtaining a second opinion causes you unnecessary stress, then do not worry about it.

More importantly, go with the doctor and the plan that gives you the most peace—the one you can best live with. Some patients prefer a teaching cancer center. Others are more comfortable at a local cancer center. Be your own advocate and go where you want to be treated.

Most doctors have only the best intentions. They use their knowledge, skills, and experience to make the most accurate diagnoses and most effective treatment recommendations. However, remember that doctors are only human and are susceptible to errors like all humanity.

A second opinion will either confirm your first diagnosis and recommended course of treatment or not. If the second confirms the first, you are likely to have peace with returning to your original doctor, prepared to proceed with the treatment plan.

When a doctor-patient relationship is no longer positive for the doctor or patient, it may be time to find another doctor with whom you feel more confident and comfortable. Ultimately, patients must be their own best advocates.

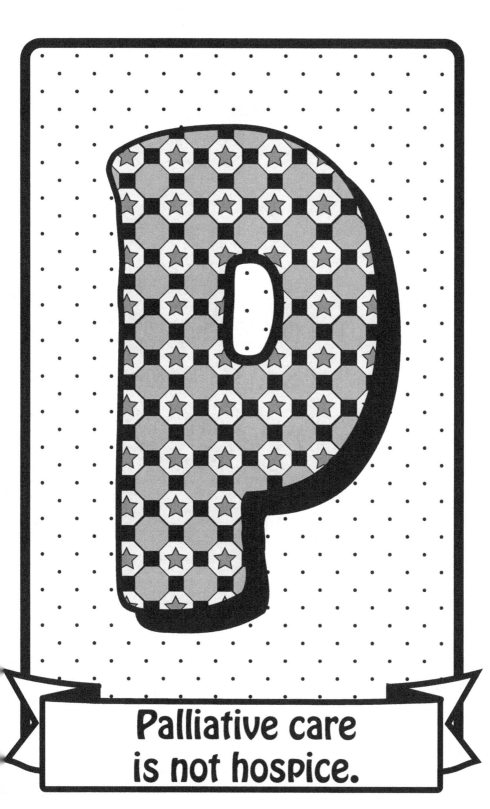

Palliative care
is not hospice.

I have come to believe that caring for myself is not self-indulgent. Caring for myself is an act of survival.
~ Audre Lorde

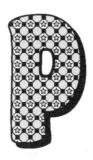

PALLIATIVE CARE IS NOT HOSPICE

There is a serious misunderstanding among cancer patients—and even health-care providers—about palliative care. What is it? Who needs it? How does it differ from hospice?

Palliative care helps prevent or relieve symptoms of cancer and treatment side effects. You can receive palliative care at any stage of illness. The goal of palliative care is to improve quality of life. It addresses issues such as pain management, nausea, and fatigue. Palliative care goes further by providing emotional support to patients. It also helps patients' families and caregivers.

Some health-care providers inadvertently withhold palliative care from patients because they, too, misunderstand the purpose of palliative care.

Sadly, many patients refuse palliative care because they mistakenly believe palliative care is end-of-life care. Furthermore, some health-care providers inadvertently withhold palliative care from patients because they, too, misunderstand the purpose of palliative care.

Many lung cancer patients and their co-survivors can benefit from palliative care. According to the American Society of Clinical Oncology (ASCO), research indicates that patients who receive palliative care alongside anticancer treatment often have fewer symptoms, maintain a better quality of life, and are more satisfied with their treatment plans.

Ideally, lung cancer patients' treatment plans include palliative care from the outset. If it turns out the patient has no need for palliative care, fine. Nevertheless, if the patient needs support to relieve symptoms or side effects, he or she is more likely to make a smooth transition into palliative care after having been introduced early on to palliative caregivers.

Hospice focuses on quality of life, also; however, hospice is generally part of end-of-life care. On the other hand, a patient can receive palliative care at any time during the cancer journey—from early stage to end of life.

The booklet *ASCO Answers: Palliative Care* makes the distinction between the two as follows: "Palliative care is given at every step of the treatment process as an extra layer of support for people with any stage of cancer. Hospice care is a specific type of palliative care provided to people with later-stage disease who are expected to live six months or less."

Whether you can benefit from palliative care or hospice care, understand that they are both offered to improve the quality of your life. And, after all, don't we all desire to have the highest quality of life possible?

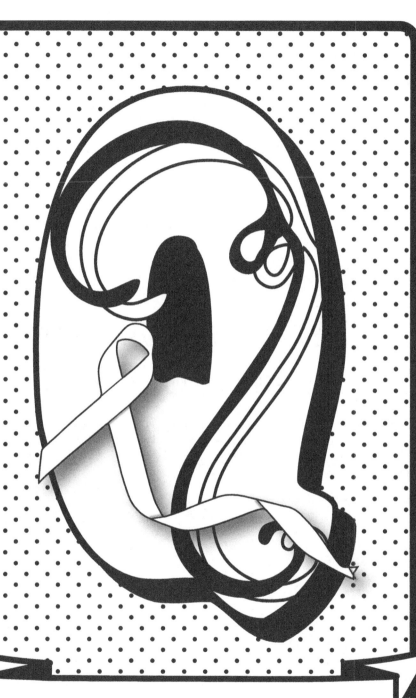

Quitting is a good idea!

To be a champ, you have to believe in yourself when nobody else will.
~ Sugar Ray Robinson

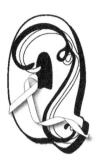

QUITTING SMOKING IS GOOD AT ANY STAGE IN YOUR LIFE

We want to shed light on this very difficult issue. We believe in approaching the topic of smoking in a positive and constructive manner that avoids ploys of fear, guilt, and condemnation. So-called public service messages about smoking have lambasted smokers. Instead of delivering antismoking messages, overzealous campaigns actually attack people who smoke. These campaigns show morbid images of people suffering from the final stages of lung cancer. Is this tactic supposed to terrorize smokers to quit or repulse others against smokers?

We understand the challenge. We believe in you.

Can you image any other disease in which horrific images try to change another's behavior? Can you image the public outcry over exploiting a person dying of AIDS because he or she had unprotected sex? Why, then, do some think it acceptable to make such an example of people dying of lung cancer? These images do far more damage than good. They increase the stigma of lung cancer patients—whether or not they have a history of smoking. We believe there is a better way.

We do not condemn smokers, nor do we condone smoking. We encourage people who want to quit to seek resources for help. Many people who smoke want to quit and have tried repeatedly, without success. However, chances for success increase with each attempt. Tools are available to help people who want to quit smoking. It is difficult but not impossible.

If you are a smoker, chances are you are around other people who also smoke. We encourage you to share information about screening with those around you who are at risk for lung cancer.

We hope you receive this message in the right spirit. We do not say this to judge or condemn. We believe lung cancer patients have to deal with far too much of that already. We understand the challenge. We believe in you.

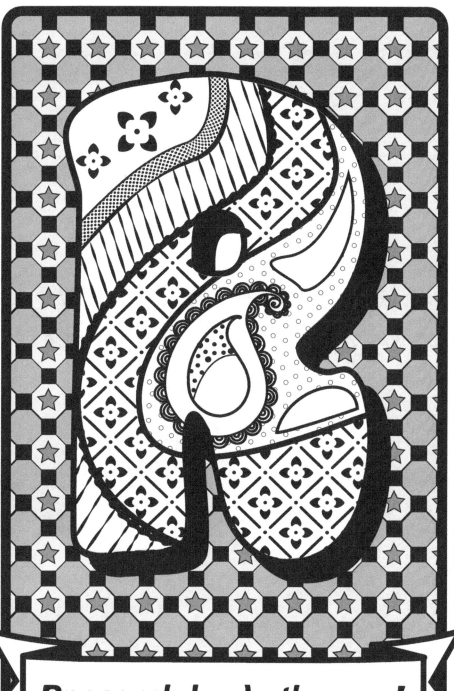

Research leads the way!

Learn from yesterday, live for today,
hope for tomorrow. The important thing
is not to stop questioning.
~Albert Einstein

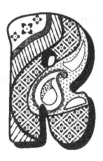

Research Is Leading the Way

We are at the dawn of a new era of lung cancer research. Literally thousands of brilliant scientists and researchers all over the world are dedicated to improving and saving the lives of people with lung cancer. Some focus on early detection; others focus on prevention, diagnosis, or treatment. Through research, we now have lung cancer screening. Recent research breakthroughs have brought targeted therapy—and, with it, a new wave of hope.

New drugs in the research pipeline hold great promise and hope for lung cancer patients.

For some patients, targeted therapy is truly a miracle. Before targeted therapy, lung cancer treatment had remained stagnant for years. But after scientists identified certain mutations in lung cancer tumor cells, they developed new anticancer drugs that strategically target and hinder the production of cancer cells. Targeted therapy has the potential to be more effective against cancer cells while being less destructive to normal cells. Personalized medicine uses intricate knowledge about an individual and his or her cancer on a cellular level to thwart new cancer growth. Even though only a small percentage of patients respond to targeted therapy, it may add quality years to the lives of those it helps.

The only way to know if an individual has a particular mutation is to test. For example, some lung cancer patients have a tumor biomarker known as epidermal growth factor receptor (EGFR). The targeted therapy known as erlotinib may be more effective in those patients with EGFR mutations. Another mutation, ALK (anaplastic lymphoma kinase), has a targeted therapy known as crizotinib.

Unfortunately, not every patient is a good candidate for targeted therapy. Because targeted therapy is relatively new, only a few identified mutations have approved treatments.

Evidence indicates another obstacle is that, eventually, cancer develops resistance to these targeted therapies.

Personalized medicine holds the promise that one day, we will have a better way to fight lung cancer. Nevertheless, for many patients, traditional chemotherapy continues to save lives.

Still, research is leading the way and making progress. Breakthroughs are happening at a faster rate than ever before. New drugs in the research pipeline hold great promise and hope for lung cancer patients. Truly, tomorrow could be the day that research changes everything—if not for everyone, then perhaps for you or your loved one.

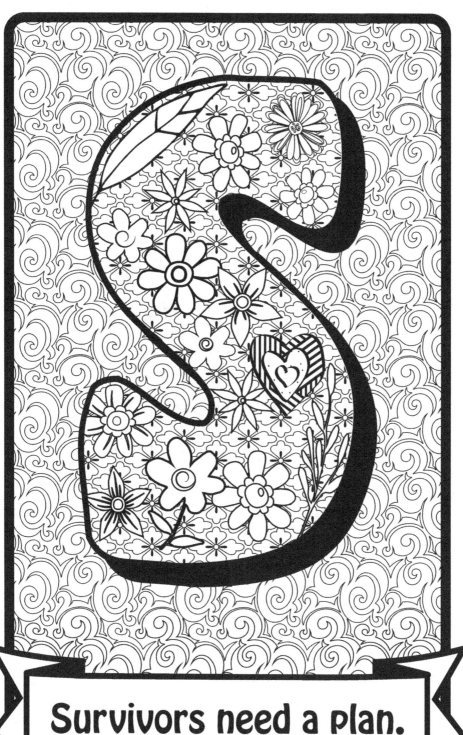

Survivors need a plan.

"For I know the plans I have for you,"
declares the Lord,
"plans to prosper you
and not to harm you,
plans to give you hope and a future."
~ Jeremiah 29:11 (NIV)

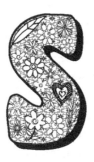

SURVIVORS NEED A PLAN

After dodging the cancer bullet, many patients feel suspended in a state of limbo, struggling with the physical and psychological aftereffects of treatment, facing fear of recurrence, and dealing with financial repercussions and unexpected challenges at work. For many cancer survivors, the future seems more uncertain than ever before.

In defining a cancer survivor, the National Cancer Institute states that "a person is considered to be a survivor from the time of diagnosis until the end of life." Some patients prefer the term "living with cancer." The National Coalition for Cancer Survivorship defines cancer survivorship as the "experience of living with, through, and beyond a diagnosis of cancer." Whatever the label, people with a history of cancer need a plan.

A survivorship plan helps patients transition from cancer patient to cancer survivor.

A survivorship plan is a complete record of a cancer patient's cancer history, treatments given, need for future checkups and cancer tests, possible long-term effects of treatment, and advice for staying healthy. The plan also identifies the health-care providers who provided care.

A survivorship plan helps patients transition from cancer

patient to cancer survivor. It also helps healthcare providers, including primary care providers and others who may not be familiar with a patient's cancer journey, understand the person's diagnosis and treatment.

Several survivorship care plans are available online, free of cost. Doctors and patients can collaborate to create customized patient-focused survivorship plans that enable patients to live healthy, active, empowered lives. Basic survivorship care plans include the following:

- Summary of diagnosis and treatment, including details about radiation, chemotherapy, and other treatments used
- Recommendations for specific action to monitor for recurrence and secondary cancers
- Risks for developing complications and long-term side effects from treatment or cancer
- Advice for living a healthy lifestyle
- Resources for employment or insurance issues, as well as psychological support services

Aside from the formal survivorship plan developed with healthcare providers, survivors may want develop their own plans based on what is important to them, such as setting meaningful life goals.

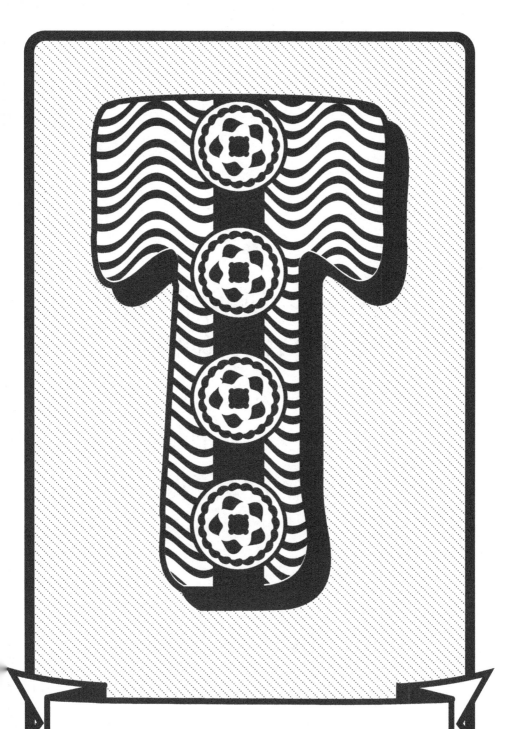

Test for radon!

Home is a sanctuary for me and
the place where I can relax.
Everyone should have the right to
a safe and secure home.
~ Corinne Bailey Rae

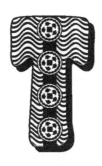

TEST YOUR HOME FOR RADON

As mentioned previously, radon is the number-two cause of lung cancer, second only to smoking. Moreover, in people who never smoked, radon is the number-one cause of lung cancer. Radon kills more than twenty thousand Americans each year, according to the Environmental Protection Agency. In fact, radon-induced lung cancer kills more Americans than drunk driving, AIDS, drowning, or home fires. We know about these other risks, but few people are aware of the risk of radon.

The only way to know if your home has high levels of radon is to test.

Radon is an odorless, invisible radioactive gas created by the naturally occurring decomposition of uranium in the soil and bedrock. Even though radon exposure is serious—potentially deadly—radon testing is inexpensive and easy. The only way to know if your home has high levels of radon is to test. Radon test kits, available at most home improvement stores, cost approximately fifteen dollars; they also are available on our website (radon.com/sub/livelung), and our nonprofit organization receives a donation from the sale.

If you detect a high radon level in your home, fixing the problem—called mitigation—is relatively inexpensive and usually takes only about a day or so, unlike remediation of other environmental hazards in the home, such as lead or mold. As with any home-improvement project, you may want to get a couple of estimates. Costs will vary depending on the size of the home and complexity of the project, but may range between $1,200 and $1,500. In some areas, financial assistance and low-interest loans are available.

January is Radon Action Month, but any time is a good time to test your home for radon. Mitigating your home increases its value. Enjoy the health benefits of testing and mitigating your home now.

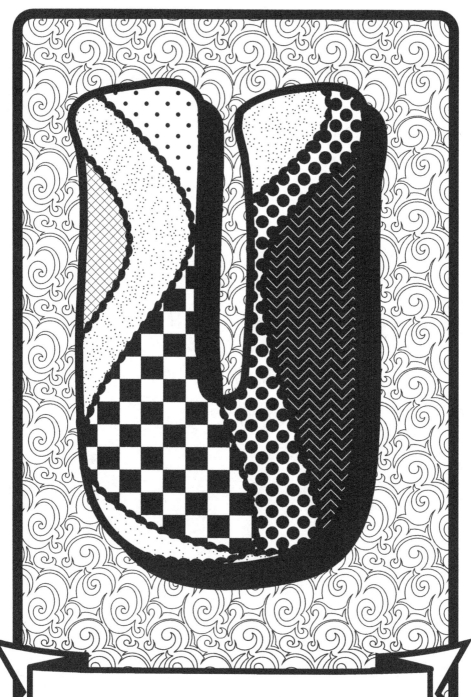

Understand your doctor.

The important thing about any word is
how you understand it.
~ Publilius Syrus

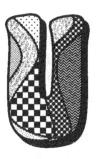

Understand What Your Doctor Says

It is very important to bring someone with you to your medical appointments for several reasons. When a patient hears, "You have lung cancer," those words may repeatedly echo in his or her mind. Those four words carry a powerful impact that takes time to absorb and comprehend. As the doctor continues speaking about important information, such as the type of lung cancer, staging, and treatment options, the patient may be unable to focus or understand what else the doctor has to say.

Write your questions in a notebook and take it with you to your appointment.

It is amazing how much information patients miss and how many of their questions go unanswered—simply because they did not ask! Inevitably, when leaving the doctor's office, a person's mind is suddenly flooded with all the questions he or she intended to ask since the last visit. It happens to more patients that you would imagine. But there is a simple solution: write your questions in a notebook that you take with you to your appointment. Make notes of the doctor's responses. Better yet, have the person with you write down the answers.

Double-check your list of questions before leaving the doctor's office. If you do not understand the doctor's explanation or instructions, tell the doctor. Do not leave that office before understanding what transpired. Some people record their conversations with their doctors—not because they don't trust their doctors, but, more likely, they don't trust their own memories, especially if they are dealing with "chemobrain," which disrupts their cognitive abilities. Your brain may have a tendency to fixate on a single statement the doctor says, such as, "Your CT scan shows new cancer growth." A statement like that can play over and over in a patient's mind as the doctor dispenses valuable information about the recommended treatment. Some doctors do not mind you recording their conversation. Some do. Use your own good judgment.

Regardless of whether or not you record the conversation, someone needs to take notes. When you leave the office, you should have a good enough understanding that you can explain to others, specifically your loved ones, what happened at your doctor's visit.

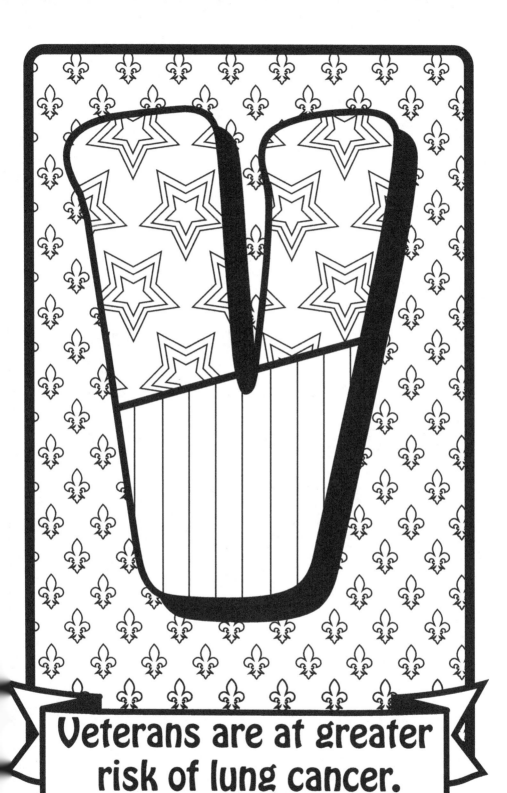

Veterans are at greater risk of lung cancer.

Our debt to the heroic men and valiant women in the service of our country can never be repaid. They have earned our undying gratitude. America will never forget their sacrifices.
~ Harry S. Truman

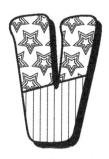

Veterans May Be at Greater Risk for Lung Cancer

Research indicates that military veterans may have a higher incidence of lung cancer and a lower survival rate compared to the general population. Our military veterans deserve greater honor rather than greater risk. However, due to exposure to potentially cancer-causing agents, military personnel and veterans are especially susceptible to lung cancer.

Our military veterans deserve greater honor rather than greater risk.

Military personnel are, or have been, exposed to chemicals known to cause lung cancer, including, but not limited to the following:

- Agent Orange
- Depleted uranium
- Diesel fuel
- Asbestos
- Ionizing radiation
- Silica

In addition to exposure to hazardous chemicals, military personnel have a higher rate of smoking history, compared to the general population, especially during wartime. Previously, the government provided cigarettes to military personnel as a standard part of their daily K-ration. They also offered deeply discounted cigarette prices to military personnel.

Now, fortunately, the Department of Defense (DoD) actually funds lung cancer research, with a particular emphasis on research that could benefit military veterans. From 2009 to 2016, the DoD funded more than one hundred million dollars in lung cancer research. The DoD seeks research projects, including environmental exposures other than tobacco, that address an aspect of lung cancer with direct relevance to military service members, veterans, and other military beneficiaries.

In addition, in September 2016, the National Cancer Institute (NCI), Department of Veterans Affairs (VA), and the DoD announced a tri-agency initiative focusing lung cancer screening in soldiers and veterans. The program, part of the federal government's Cancer Moonshot initiative, aims to boost enrollment in clinical trials to hasten new targeted treatments. VA medical centers will expand their participation in NCI's network of clinical trial sites and partner with other sponsors of clinical trials testing targeted therapies. This will improve veterans' access to new therapies through clinical trials. These initiatives give veterans more reasons to hope.

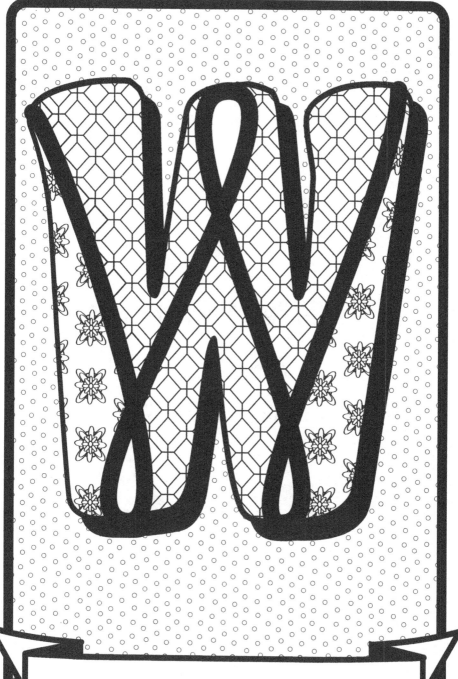

Write your story.

Writing is the art of making people real to themselves with words.

~ Logan Pearsall Smith

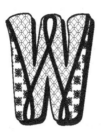

Write Your Story

Everyone has a story. Too often, compelling stories go untold. Writing can be a way to capture and express your lung cancer journey. It can be therapeutic. It can encourage and comfort others. It can give an accurate account of your life. Writing can be an outlet for thoughts and feelings that you may be uncomfortable expressing verbally. You may understand your own story better after writing it down. There are as many reasons to write as there are words to write.

Writing can be a way to capture and express your lung cancer journey.

Don't think you have to have it all organized in your mind before you start writing—just write! You can organize it after you jot down your thoughts. If an outline helps you fill in the blanks, do that. Do whatever works best for you.

Start small. Try writing three words to describe someone you encountered previously in the week. Then write three words that describe you. Next, write what you felt when you were told you have lung cancer, whether a full page, a few paragraphs, or a few sentences. Try to freeze that moment in your mind. Write descriptively. Look around and note every sensation—what you see and how it makes you feel. Make it personal.

Your story is not an accumulation of medical facts and procedures. Resist the urge to get bogged down in treatment details—how many radiation treatments you had, side effects of your chemo, neuropathy, and so on. Frankly, because those are experiences others may not be able to relate to, most readers will lose interest in treatment specifics. Even though you may have endured a great deal of suffering during treatment, keep those details brief in your writing. If you feel compelled to go into details about your treatment, do so in another document that is separate from your personal story. A perfect time to share those details is at a lung cancer support group or advocacy meeting, when you are among other lung cancer patients. These stories will intrigue other lung cancer patients.

After you write it, practice speaking it. You will become more comfortable sharing one on one and in a group setting. Sharing your personal story will help further the cause of lung cancer awareness.

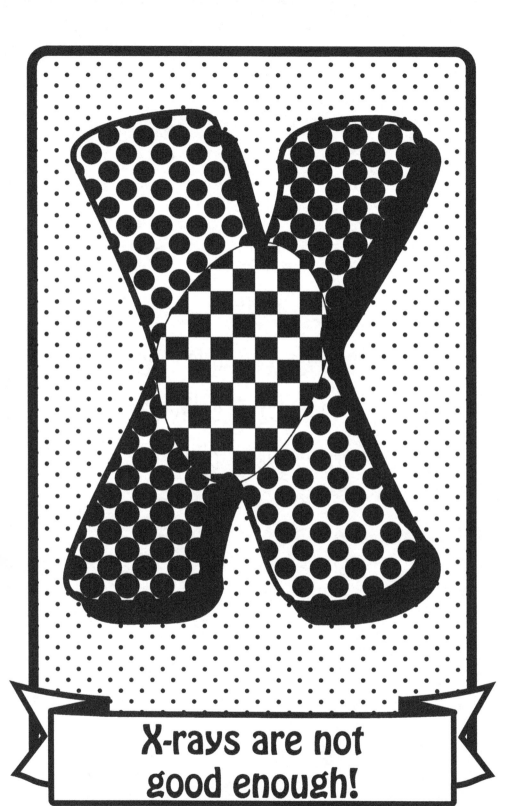

X-rays are not
good enough!

Whoever saves a life, it is considered
as if he saved an entire world.
~ Yerushalmi Talmud 4:9

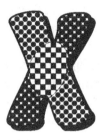

X-RAYS ARE NOT GOOD ENOUGH!

A CT scan is the most effective way to detect lung cancer early. After dismal decades with no early detection for the number-one cancer killer, a major research project changed everything. The National Lung Screening Trial decisively proved that lung cancer screening by annual low-dose CT scans reduces lung cancer's mortality rate by 20 percent.

Medicare and Medicaid also cover lung cancer screening, in large part due to the efforts of the lung cancer community.

The study involved more than fifty-three thousand Americans identified as high risk for lung cancer based on two criteria: age and smoking history. The minimum age was fifty-five, and the minimum smoking history was thirty pack years. (As mentioned previously, calculate pack years by multiplying the number of cigarette packs the person smoked per day by the number of years the person smoked. For example, someone who smoked two packs a day for fifteen years has a thirty-pack-year smoking history.) Former smokers who quit smoking within the previous fifteen years also enrolled in the study.

Half of the participants, more than twenty-six thousand, were randomly assigned annual screening by chest x-rays. The other half were screened by low-dose CT scans. The group screened by low-dose CT scans showed a 20 percent decreased mortality rate compared with those screened by chest x-rays.

For those who meet the age and smoking-history guidelines, private insurance companies often cover lung cancer screening with no copay or out-of-pocket cost to the patient. Medicare and Medicaid also cover lung cancer screening, in large part due to the efforts of the lung cancer community. (After receiving advocates' responses, authorities reversed their initial recommendation against covering screening.)

Lung cancer screening by low-dose CT scans is fast and painless. Because CT scans can detect even a tiny nodule, a common problem with the procedure is a high rate of "false positives," nodules that ultimately prove to be harmless. Understanding this risk prior to being screened may help reduce unnecessary anxiety. The high false-positive rate is one of the reasons insurers require a shared decision-making discussion about the risks and benefits of screening by low-dose CT.

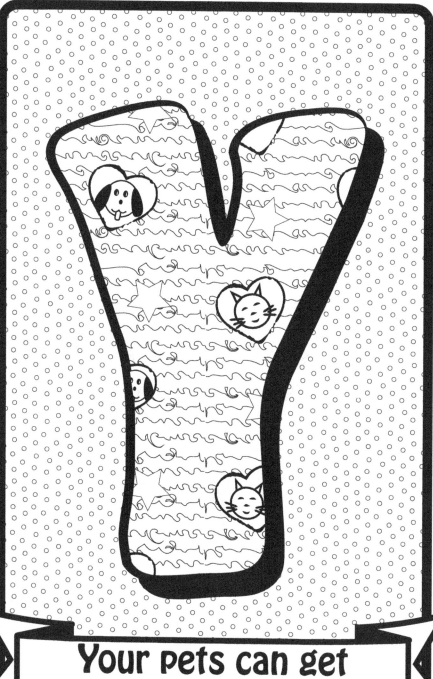

Your pets can get lung cancer, too.

A righteous man (or woman) cares for
the needs of his animal...
Proverbs 12:10 (NIV)

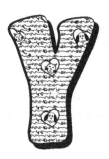

Your Pet Can Get Lung Cancer, Too

Our four-legged children have lungs and are subject to some of the same environmental hazards as we are. Radon is a risk factor for dogs and cats, too. Radon is heavier than air, so usually in a home with high radon, it is more concentrated closer to the floor, where our pets hang out. Animals can develop lung cancer from radon and from secondhand smoke.

One of the activities our nonprofit organization does is distribute radon test kits in high radon communities. During one such event, a man told me he had lost five dogs to lung cancer. I do not know what his test result revealed, but I strongly suspect his home had high radon.

Since we are talking about animals, another passion of mine, an additional important pet-related topic is arranging for their care when you are no longer able to care for them. My husband and I have worked with rescue organizations and have been surprised—and deeply saddened—at the number of pets abandoned after their owners pass away. Far too often, when a loved one dies, the person's pet is treated like a used mattress. Animals that were greatly loved by their owners are abandoned or dumped at shelters. The lucky ones may find another home. Many,

Ask someone special in your life to adopt your pet when your time comes.

however, will live the remainder of their days in shelters, grieving for their owners and longing for human love—or, worse, be put down.

Ask someone special in your life to adopt your pet when your time comes. Let others know about arrangements for your pet. Do not assume your animals will be taken care of. Please prepare for their care.

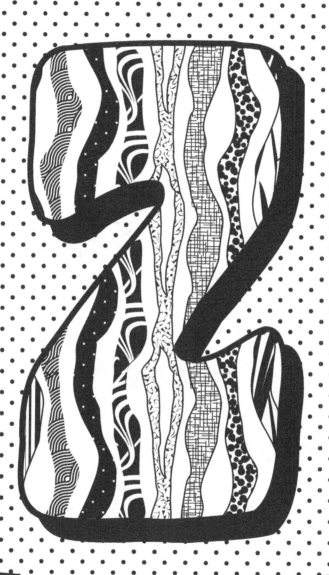

Zealously advocate!

The only thing necessary for the triumph of evil is for good men (and women) to do nothing.
~ Edmund Burke

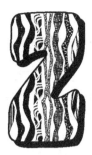

ZEALOUSLY ADVOCATE FOR YOURSELF AND OTHERS

- You can advocate in small ways or go all out.
- Share information about early detection with a lung cancer-screening candidate. You may just save a life!
- Write and share your story. Write a letter about lung cancer awareness to the editor of your local newspaper.
- Develop your survivorship plan.
- Give the gift of time or money to support a nonprofit organization serving the lung cancer community.

The most important thing for a lung cancer patient to do is simply be well.

- Make your final wishes known, including plans for your pets.
- Keep lung cancer symptoms and warning signs in mind and let your doctor know of any new developments. Remember to make your list of questions and take someone with you to appointments. Ask the doctor to repeat instructions or clarify anything you do not understand. Ask your doctor if a clinical trial might be right for you.
- Enlighten others about the stigma of lung cancer and the disparity of research funding.
- Please do not forget to test your home for radon. Give radon test kits as stocking stuffers to your loved ones.

These ABCs of lung cancer are simply the beginning. Build on this foundation to increase your knowledge and become an effective advocate. God knows we need you. If you are going through treatment, breathe easy. The most important thing for a lung cancer patient to do is simply be well. If any of these advocacy activities brings you stress, then delegate. The next time someone offers to help, share this book with him or her. If, on the other hand, being a lung cancer advocate enriches and empowers your life, then, by all means, do it!

ABOUT THE AUTHORS

Dusty Joy Donaldson became a lung cancer advocate immediately following her lung cancer diagnosis in September 2005. She volunteered with several nonprofit organizations for approximately five years. In 2010, with the support of her husband Tony and her children, Kimberly, Kirk and Amy, Dusty founded the Dusty Joy Foundation (dba LiveLung), a 501(c)(3) with a mission of advancing lung cancer awareness, early detection and compassion for people impacted by lung cancer. She is co-leader of the Lung Cancer Action Network (LungCAN). Prior to her diagnosis, Dusty was a journalist at daily newspapers in Virginia and North Carolina. She earned several journalism awards from the Virginia Press Association. She later became a communications and media relations specialist. She earned a BA in journalism from Norfolk State University in Norfolk, Virginia and an MA in public policy journalism from Regent University in Virginia Beach, Virginia. She also earned a certificate in Nonprofit Management from Duke University. Dusty lives in High Point, North Carolina, with her husband and their four rescue kitties: Boots, Xena, Buttons and Butterscotch.

Kimberly D. Lester became a lung cancer advocate after her mother's lung cancer diagnosis in 2005. Since then she has devoted much of her free time supporting the lung cancer cause through social media, artistic designs, charity events and many other ways. Her creative skillsets in the areas of writing and design have proven valuable in elevating awareness. Kimberly contributes to the day-to-day activities of the Dusty Joy Foundation and LungCAN while holding a fulltime position. Currently, she is a Technical Writer at Jenzabar in Harrisonburg, Virginia. Kimberly earned a BS in Professional Writing from Old Dominion University in Virginia. She lives in the Shenandoah Valley with her husband Kirk and a kitty who sleeps all day. Her adult son, Jacob, lives nearby.

REFERENCES AND RESOURCES

Links posted at LiveLung.org/ABCs.

A

National Institutes of Health's National Cancer Institute (NIH's NCI). "Surveillance, Epidemiology and End Results Program: SEER Stat Fact Sheets: Lung and Bronchus Cancer." Accessed October 12, 2016. http://www.seer.cancer.gov/statfacts/html/lungb.html.

U.S. Environmental Protection Agency (EPA). "Radon." Accessed October 12, 2016. http://www.epa.gov/radon.

EPA. "Health Risk of Radon." Accessed October 12, 2016. http://www.epa.gov/radon/health-risk-radon.

EPA. "A Citizens Guide to Radon" (page 2)." Accessed October 12, 2016. https://www.epa.gov/sites/production/files/2016-02/documents/2012_a_citizens_guide_to_radon.pdf.

American Cancer Society (ACS). "Why Non-smokers Sometimes Get Lung Cancer." October 30, 2015. Accessed October 12, 2016. http://www.cancer.org/cancer/news/features/why-lung-cancer-strikes-nonsmokers.

MacReady, Norra. "Many Lung Cancer Patients Stopped Smoking Years Before Diagnosis." (Poster 4 Presented at the 11th International Lung Cancer Conference. July 10, 2010. http://www.medscape.com/viewarticle/725138.

B

ACS. "Signs and Symptoms of Lung Cancer." Accessed October 12, 2016. www.cancer.org/cancer/lungcancer-non-smallcell/moreinformation/lungcancerpreventionandearlydetection/lung-cancer-prevention-and-early-detection-signs-and-symptoms.

C

NIH. "Clinical Trials." Accessed October 12, 2016. https://clinicaltrials.gov.

EmergingMed. "Clinical Trial Navigation Service." Accessed October 12, 2016. https://www.emergingmed.com.

NIH NCI. "Clinical Trials Information for Patients and Caregivers." Accessed October 12, 2016. https://www.cancer.gov/about-cancer/treatment/clinical-trials.

D

A Chapple. "Stigma, Shame, And Blame Experienced By Patients With Lung Cancer: Qualitative Study." *British Medical Journal.* (June 17, 2004.) Accessed October 12, 2016. www.bmj.com/content/328/7454/1470.

Brigham and Women's Hospital. "Out of the Shadows: Women and Lung Cancer." (May 2010.) Accessed October 12, 2016. www.brighamandwomens.org/departments_and_services/womenshealth/connorscenter/images/womenandlungcancerfinal-april22,2010pdf.pdf.

E

U.S. Preventive Services Task Force. "Lung Cancer: Screening." (December 2013) Accessed October 12, 2016. www.uspreventiveservicestaskforce.org/Page/Document/UpdateSummaryFinal/lung-cancer-screening.

National Comprehensive Cancer Network (NCCN). "NCCN Guidelines for Patients: Lung Cancer Screening." (January 2016) Accessed October 12, 2016. www.nccn.org/patients/guidelines/lung_screening/index.html.

Centers for Medicare and Medicaid Services. "Decision Memo for Screening for Lung Cancer with Low Dose Computed Tomography."(February 5, 2015) Accessed October 12, 2016. www.cms.gov/medicare-coverage-database/details/nca-decision-memo.aspx?NCAId=274.

F

ACS. "Surveillance and Health Services Research." (2014) Accessed October 12, 2016. www.cancer.org/acs/groups/content/@research/documents/document/a cspc-042801.pdf

G

Dusty Joy Foundation (LiveLung). "What Your Gift Can Do" Accessed October 12, 2016. www.livelung.org/donate.

LiveLung. "Want to Help?" Accessed October 12, 2016. www.livelung.org/resources/want-to-help.

H

U.S. Congress. "Recalcitrant Cancer Research Act." Accessed October 12, 2016. https://www.congress.gov/bill/112th-congress/house-bill/733.

I

Wikipedia. "List of Awareness Ribbons." (Page modified October 6, 2016.) Accessed October 12, 2016. https://en.wikipedia.org/wiki/List_of_awareness_ribbons.

Lung Cancer Alliance (LCA). "About." Accessed October 12, 2016. www.lungcanceralliance.org/about-lca.

J

LiveLung. "Lung Cancer Support Groups." Accessed October 12, 2016. www.livelung.org/community/support-group-meetings.

LCA. "Lung Cancer Support Groups." Accessed October 12, 2016. www.lungcanceralliance.org/get-help-and-support/coping-with-lung-cancer/support-groups.

K

NIH NCI Surveillance, Epidemiology and End Results Program. "SEER Stat Fact Sheets: Lung and Bronchus Cancer." Accessed October 12, 2016. www.seer.cancer.gov/statfacts/html/lungb.html

EPA. "Radon Health Risks." Accessed October 12, 2016. https://www.epa.gov/radon/health-risk-radon.

L

LiveLung. "Charlotte's Story." Accessed October 12, 2016. www.livelung.org/testimonials_slides/charlottes-story.

WikiHow. "How to Make Your Bucket List." Accessed October 12, 2016. www.wikihow.com/Make-Your-Bucket-List.

M

U.S. Department of Health & Human Services's National Institute on Aging. "Health & Aging: Getting Your Affairs in Order." Accessed October 12, 2016. www.nia.nih.gov/health/publication/getting-your-affairs-order.

NCCN. "Patient and Caregiver Resources: Advance Directives." Accessed October 12, 2016. www.nccn.org/patients/resources/life_with_cancer/advance_directives.aspx.

N

Lanford, Julie. Cancer Dietician. Accessed October 12, 2016. www.cancerdietitian.com.

O

Patient Advocate Foundation. "Second Opinions." Accessed October 12, 2016. www.patientadvocate.org/help.php/index.php?p=691.

ACS. "Seeking a Second Opinion." Accessed October 12, 2016. www.cancer.org/treatment/findingandpayingfortreatment/seeking-a-second-opinion.

P

American Society of Clinical Oncologists (ASCO). "Palliative Care." Accessed October 12, 2016. www.cancer.net/navigating-cancer-care/how-cancer-treated/palliative-care.

ASCO. "ACSO Answers: Palliative Care." Accessed October 12, 2016. www.cancer.net/sites/cancer.net/files/palliative_care.pdf.

NIH NCI. "Palliative Care in Cancer." Accessed October 12, 2016. https://www.cancer.gov/about-cancer/advanced-cancer/care-choices/palliative-care-fact-sheet.

Q

Quit Smoking Community. Accessed October 12, 2016. https://quitsmokingcommunity.org.

R

International Association for the Study of Lung Cancer (IASLC). Accessed October 12, 2016. www.iaslc.org.

ASCO. "Research & Progress." Accessed October 12, 2016. www.asco.org/research-progress.

EmergingMed. Accessed October 12, 2016. www.emergingmed.com.

S

LiveStrong Foundation. "LiveStrong Care Plan." Accessed October 12, 2016. www.livestrongcareplan.org.

ASCO. "ASCO Cancer Treatment and Survivorship Care Plans." Accessed October 12, 2016. www.cancer.net/survivorship/follow-care-after-cancer-treatment/asco-cancer-treatment-and-survivorship-care-plans.

National Coalition for Cancer Survivorship (NCCS). Accessed October 12, 2016. www.canceradvocacy.org.

T

Kansas State University National Radon Program Services. Accessed October 12, 2016. www.sosradon.org.

EPA. "Radon." Accessed October 12, 2016. www.epa.gov/radon.

USDHHS. "Healthfinder: Test Your Home for Radon: Quick Tips." Accessed October 12, 2016. www.healthfinder.gov/healthtopics/category/pregnancy/getting-ready-for-your-baby/test-your-home-for-radon-quick-tips.

LiveLung.org. "Order Kit." Accessed October 12, 2016. www.livelung.org/radon-red/order-kit.

U

NCCS. "Communicating with Your Doctor." Accessed October 12, 2016. www.canceradvocacy.org/resources/communicating-with-your-doctor.

CancerCare. "'Doctor, Can We Talk?': Tips for Communicating With Your Health Care Team." Accessed October 12, 2016. www.cancercare.org/publications/53-doctor_can_we_talk_tips_for_communicating_with_your_health_care_team.

Family Caregiver Alliance. "Communicating with Your Doctor." Accessed October 12, 2016. www.caregiver.org/communicating-your-doctor.

ASCO. "ASCO Answers: Non-Small Cell Lung Cancer." Accessed October 12, 2016. www.cancer.net/sites/cancer.net/files/asco_answers_guide_nsclc.pdf.

ASCO. "ASCO Answers: Small Cell Lung Cancer, American Society of Clinical Oncology." Accessed October 12, 2016. www.cancer.net/sites/cancer.net/files/asco_answers_guide_sclc.pdf

V

Veterans News Now. "Higher Rates of Lung Cancer Among Gulf War, Other Veterans." Accessed October 13, 2016. www.veteransnewsnow.com/2012/04/23/higher-rates-of-lung-cancer-among-gulf-war-other-veterans-immediate-medical-research-funding-availability-through-cdmrp.

U.S. Department of Defense. "Congressionally Directed Medical Research Program: Lung Cancer." Accessed October 13, 2016. http://cdmrp.army.mil/lcrp.

Department of Veterans Affairs. "Tri-Agency Partnership Working to Tailor Cancer Care Based on Genes, Proteins." Accessed October 13, 2016. http://www.va.gov/opa/pressrel/pressrelease.cfm?id=2810.

The White House. "Fact Sheet: Investing in the National Cancer Moonshot." Accessed October 13, 2016. https://www.whitehouse.gov/the-press-office/2016/02/01/fact-sheet-investing-national-cancer-moonshot.

W

Ness, RN, Sheryl M. "Cancer Survivors Take Control by Writing Their Own Story." Mayo Clinic. Accessed October 13, 2016. www.mayoclinic.org/diseases-conditions/cancer/expert-blog/writing-your-cancer-story/bgp-20138991.

Evans, John, MAT, MA, EdD. "Legacy Writing." Survivor's Review. Accessed October 13, 2016. www.survivorsreview.org/writenow.php

Solomon, Michael. "Let It Out: Writing About Your Cancer." I Had Cancer. Accessed October 13, 2016. www.ihadcancer.com/h3-blog/12-14-2012/let-it-out-writing-about-your-cancer.

X

National Lung Screening Trial Research Team. "Reduced Lung-Cancer Mortality with Low-Dose Computed Tomographic Screening." *New England Journal of Medicine.* (August 4, 2010) Accessed October 13, 2016. www.nejm.org/doi/full/10.1056/NEJMoa1102873.

U.S. Preventive Services Task Force. "Lung Cancer: Screening." Accessed October 13, 2016. www.uspreventiveservicestaskforce.org/Page/Document/UpdateSummary Final/lung-cancer-screening.

NCCN. "NCCN Guidelines for Patients: Lung Cancer Screening." January 2016. Accessed October 13, 2016. www.nccn.org/patients/guidelines/lung_screening/index.html.

Centers for Medicare and Medicaid Services. "Decision Memo for Screening for Lung Cancer with Low Dose Computed Tomography." February 5, 2015. Accessed October 13, 2016. www.cms.gov/medicare-coverage-database/details/nca-decision-memo.aspx?NCAId=274.

Y

Renzulli, Kerri Anne. "How to Make Sure Your Pet Is Cared for When You Die." *Money Magazine.* Accessed October 13, 2016. www.time.com/money/4110085/pet-trust-estate-planning.

Millan, Cesar. "Dog In Mourning: Helping Our Pets Cope with Loss." Cesar's Way. Accessed October 13, 2016. www.cesarsway.com/dog-behavior/problem-behaviors/a-dog-in-mourning-helping-our-pets-cope.

Krieger, Marilyn. "7 Ways to Help Your Cat Through a Grieving Period." Catster. Accessed October 13, 2016. www.catster.com/lifestyle/cat-behavior-tips-grieving-grief.

Syufy, Franny. "The Feline-Human Bond of Love: What Happens When One Party Departs?" Accessed October 13, 2016. www.cats.about.com/cs/felinehumanbond/a/love_3.htm.

Humane Society. "Providing for Your Pet's Future without You." Accessed October 13, 2016. humanesociety.org/animals/resources/tips/providing_for_pets_future_wit hout_you.html.

Shever, Amy. "The Importance of Selecting Potential Caregivers for Your Pets." Accessed October 13, 2016. www.2ndchance4pets.org/help.html

ADDITIONAL RESOURCES

The following organizations are members of the
Lung Cancer Action Network (LungCAN).

Bonnie J. Addario Lung Cancer Foundation
lungcancerfoundation.org

CancerCare
www.cancercare.org

Cancer Support Community
www.cancersupportcommunity.org

Cancer Survivors Against Radon
(CanSAR)
www.cansar.org

Citizens for Radioactive Radon Reduction
www.citizensforradioactiveradonreduction.org

Dusty Joy Foundation (LiveLung)
www.livelung.org

Free Me from Lung Cancer
www.freemefromlungcancer.org

Free to Breathe
www.freetobreathe.org

John Atkinson Foundation
www.johnatkinsonfoundation.org

Lung Cancer Action Network
www.lungcan.org

Lung Cancer Alliance
www.lungcanceralliance.org

Lung Cancer Caring Ambassadors
www.lungcancercap.org

Lung Cancer Circle of Hope
lungcancercircleofhope.org

Lung Cancer Foundation of America
www.lcfamerica.org

LUNGevity
www.lungevity.org

Lung Force
www.lungforce.org

Lung Cancer Initiative of North Carolina
www.lungcancerinitiativenc.org

Lung Cancer Research Foundation
www.lungcancerresearchfoundation.org

Respiratory Health Association
www.lungchicago.org

Rexanna's Foundation
www.rexannasfoundation.org

Upstage Lung Cancer
upstagelungcancer.org

NOTES

_____

_____

_____

_____

_____

_____

_____

_____

_____

_____

_____

_____

_____

_____

_____

_____

_____

_____

_____

_____

_____

_____

_____

_____

NOTES

NOTES

NOTES

Made in the USA
Monee, IL
30 April 2025

16593823R00075